Overcome The BS of MS

A 3-Step Plan For Women Living With Multiple Sclerosis

By Lisa Cohen

www.rockstarwomenwithms.com

Dedication

To Donald Cohen, my beloved father, whose immeasurable love and support have helped me not only through life with MS, but throughout my entire life. Love you, Dad.

Acknowledgments

Many thanks to all of the wonderful family, friends, and kind strangers who have encouraged and supported me in my efforts to live an active life with MS and to help other women living with MS to do the same. I'm not listing names here because I'd hate to accidentally leave anyone out, and some of you have been anonymous helpful angels who happened to appear at just the right times over the years. You all know who you are. Thank you.

And many thanks to my new P'N'P family for all of your advice, support and enthusiasm (even in the wee hours of the morning). You guys are awesome.

Table of Contents

Introduction

"Sub-cutaneous...sub-cutaneous..." The word reverberated in my head while my neurologist continued speaking about the medications that were thankfully now available. *"Wait a minute,"* I said when the word finally hit home... *"NEEDLES???" "Yes,"* he said. *"Isn't there a pill that I could take?,"* I whined. Of course, the answer to that was NO. Figures.

So, there I was, more concerned about the method of medication delivery (I'm scared of needles) than about the fact that I had just been diagnosed with Multiple Sclerosis ("MS"). Seems warped, but that's how it went. Sure, I was distraught about the diagnosis, but the truth is that I felt more relieved that I didn't have something worse...It wasn't the rheumatoid arthritis that my mother had struggled with or the scleroderma that ultimately took her life in just a few short years. The way that I saw it, perhaps I might be fortunate to have a "least of the evils" situation happening.

Still, it was definitely a wrench in the works, to say the least. I had jumped ship and "escaped" the lawyer job that I hated at a big firm downtown only 4 years earlier, and had really come into my own building a great new life in the independent music business and pursuing photography. Getting sick was so not part of the plan. I had just taken the first steps toward getting my life together, and was it now all going to be snatched away? What was going to happen next? I cried in my neurologist's office.

That was the start of what would be my continuing journey of being faced with, adapting to, and managing life with what I refer to as the "BS[1] of MS"—The life changes that result from having MS and all of the physical, psychological, and emotional "stuff" that comes along with living with MS. And, let me tell you, it has been a long roller coaster ride of ups and downs...

I eventually chose what I call a "rockstar" path (you'll learn more about this whole "rockstar" terminology later in the book), but the truth is that I didn't start out that way. In fact, I did the exact opposite: I ran and hid after I was first diagnosed. I assumed that the dreams I'd been pursuing at the time of my diagnosis were over, and I made decisions for several years based on letting my MS symptoms run the show and a fear of when and how my condition would worsen, even though I hadn't yet become physically disabled. I voluntarily relegated myself to the position of backup singer in my own life while letting MS take center stage for many years, and there were many times when I let the "BS of MS" defeat me, sometimes even for several years at a time. I spent many years just passively "living small" in what felt like a "safer" yet less-than life; and I felt stuck settling for that because I was so tired (both physically from the MS and psychologically), I didn't truly believe that I had an alternative, and the truth is that it can feel just plain "easier" to give in to inertia than to change.

But, that wasn't truly me and I knew it. I had always been a high-achiever, and I still had a desire to do something that I considered "great" with my life, even if nobody knew I'd done it or considered it "great" but me...I decided to start breaking out of that "backup singer" dynamic. However, just when I'd finally broken out of it and begun taking steps to pursue a dream life again, I was abruptly knocked down by the back-to-back quintuple-whammy of being laid off when my employer collapsed at the start of the 2008 financial crisis, becoming disabled by my MS for the first time right on the heels of the layoff, experiencing an ankle injury that wouldn't heal properly for years, facing additional painful events in my personal life, and being set back for many months by a negative reaction to a new medication. I felt physically afraid, I lost my self-confidence, I lost myself, and I basically kind of gave up. Once again, I became a backup singer in my own life while letting the BS of MS run the show.

Living like that felt awful and took a huge psychological and emotional toll on me. I realized that life was passing me by, and I eventually got so fed up that I knew I had to defeat that dynamic of playing "backup singer" to the BS of MS forever. I honestly didn't know if I even had the strength in me anymore to rise above the most recent knockdowns, but I knew that I had to try. I knew that I had to start creating what felt like a rockstar life for myself again in the way that I had when I'd first risked leaving my law firm before my MS diagnosis. Sure, certain things wouldn't be or look quite the same because of my changed physical condition, but I believed that I could certainly get things to FEEL the same in the sense of actively creating a life that I chose that was a match for my personality—and that's what I define as "rockstar."

When I finally got fed-up enough, I simply began taking action to change my situation, reclaim my power, and start actively creating my life anew despite the BS of MS. Thanks to the support of amazing family and friends, I was able to do that.

Today, I rock a cane with an animal-print or sparkly cover (depending on my mood), take photographs and create art, knit teddy bears for sick and underprivileged children, am getting better at playing the guitar, and founded Rockstar Women With MS to fulfill a life purpose of helping other women with MS to live their own version of a "rockstar" life rather than succumbing to the BS of MS.

What I've learned from my own personal journey is that I have a lot more power in what happens next in my life than I'd previously believed. I've written this book for a couple of reasons. First, it's the type of support resource that I wish I'd been able to find years ago to help me actively manage the BS of MS in a way that could help me to live an active and empowered life rather than a merely "stable" (that's one of the medical buzzwords for us, which is intended to mean keeping us from getting worse, but the psychological translation of that for me equates to "stagnant" without hope of improvement) one. Second, to show women who are newly-diagnosed with MS that they don't have to take the "cut and run" option that I first did, and to show women who have played "second fiddle" to their MS—even if it's been for years—that they don't have to continue to do so. We CAN maintain or reclaim center stage and create our own rockstar lives while we are living with MS. I know that because I created and used a system that successfully allowed me to do that for myself. And, in my own experience, I found that a fundamental requirement for doing so is learning how to overcome the BS of MS, so that's what this book is about.

So, how can this book help you? Although I have created comprehensive and customized programs to provide in-depth lessons and support for overcoming the BS of MS, those take time to complete; and I realized from my own personal experience that sometimes you just need something to help get you taking action *quickly* in order to feel better right away, start seeing some tangible immediate progress, and start building some forward momentum. Let's face it, sometimes you just need the answer to *"Hey, what can I do RIGHT NOW?"* Sometimes that's an answer to the *"What do I do first?"* question, sometimes it's a simple kick-start, and sometimes it's a quick solution to the *"Help, I'm stuck"* problem. This book is designed to be an easy-read reference handbook that provides all three of those solutions to help you get started quickly on the first steps to managing the BS of MS and creating a life that you love. You can keep it nearby in your bag or on a mobile device and refer back to it whenever you feel stuck or need a bit of a pep talk.

Inside, you will find some key tools in the form of a 3-Step Plan that I personally used and continue to use to manage the BS of MS and to either prevent getting stuck in the first place or to get unstuck quickly when I need to. The 3-Step Plan is a system that you can: 1) Use to immediately start taking action (and feel better right away because you *are* taking action), 2) Turn to if you're feeling overwhelmed, 3) Use to help you get unstuck if you're currently stuck, and 4) Use to support yourself in maintaining or recharging a positive headspace so that you can continue to move forward in creating the life that you want.

Ideally, this book will save you from reinventing the wheel or falling into the same holes and traps that I did when I first started down my own path to creating a rockstar life while facing the BS of MS. As an added bonus, throughout the book, you will be given opportunities to access more in-depth resources to help you overcome the BS of MS and transform your life, and to connect with the support of a global community of rockstar women living with MS.

Best wishes and much love to you in overcoming the BS of MS and starting to create rockstar changes in your life!

JOIN US!

CONNECT WITH OUR FREE SUPPORT COMMUNITY

AT ROCKSTAR WOMEN WITH MS

and find resources to help you

overcome the BS of MS!

For a FREE BACKSTAGE PASS

and access to other cool goodies as soon as they're released,

visit www.rockstarwomenwithms.com

ONE

Who Is This Book For?

This book is for any woman who wants to truly feel like she is actively living and enjoying a life that she chooses, even though she also happens to be living with MS; and it's designed to help you start feeling that way quickly. You may have picked up this book for any number of reasons. You may have been struggling under the weight of all the BS that comes along with your MS for a long time now, and are looking for solutions to help you manage it on a daily basis. You may be feeling like you're sitting in the backseat in life while your MS is in the driver's seat and finally be completely fed up with that, or you may simply be concerned about the possibility of that happening to you in the future. Or you may feel that you don't "fit" the traditional avatar of "the person living with MS" and are feeling dissatisfied with the options for "life with MS" that you've been able to find so far. Any and all of you may be looking for some kind of system that can help you to prevail over the BS of MS on a consistent and continuing basis.

If any of these words resonate with you, then you are definitely in the right place because this book is for YOU.

To each and all of you above, I can honestly say that I totally "get" it because I've been where you are. I've experienced the shock, fear, and uncertainty of having my life rocked by an unexpected MS diagnosis as well as disability and injury. I understand the extra challenges involved in dealing with the BS of MS day-to-day and trying to create any kind of consistency while facing very real physical limitations and symptoms that fluctuate. I know what it's like to feel buried under the weight of all the BS of MS and just passively give up for a while because of sheer exhaustion. And I am also all-too-familiar with what it's like to feel just plain "stuck" in life in general and not know what to do next or how to get moving.

Because I became a firsthand expert at creating my own rockstar life before my MS diagnosis, and I then had to become a firsthand expert at managing the BS of MS out of necessity in order to create a new rockstar life after MS-related physical losses, I've written this book for you in order to to help you to do the same thing. I'm committed to helping you to create the life that you want in spite of the BS of MS that you may be facing.

So, let's get this party started…

TWO

A "BS of MS" Primer

Before we get to the 3-Step Plan, let's cover some fundamentals. Those of you living with MS probably know many facts about the disease and are likely to be quite familiar with the BS of MS already, but I felt that it might be helpful to give a quick overview for those of you without MS who may be reading this book in order to find ways to better help loved ones who are living with MS.

Multiple Sclerosis is a chronic, often disabling disease that attacks the central nervous system, which is made up of the brain, spinal cord, and optic nerves. There are approximately 400,000 people with MS in the United States today, and MS is thought to affect more than 2.1 million people worldwide.[2] MS "[t]hreatens personal autonomy, independence, dignity, and future plans. As a relapsing-remitting disorder patients face an unpredictable course; as an incurable progressive disease patients have to respond to multiple new setbacks

over time."[3] MS is typically diagnosed in the "prime" of life and is at

least 2–3 times more common in women than men.[4]   It causes

disruptions in daily routines, social lives, relationships, and

employment.   "At the moment of being diagnosed, the patient is

forever transformed into a 'person living with MS.'   Even in the

absence of signs or symptoms, this person will forever after live with

the knowledge that he or she can be unpredictably impaired.

Sometimes the person will recover, sometimes not. For most, living

with MS will become one of the major challenges of life. People with

MS need to solve problems ranging from finding the right button hook,

to getting dressed every morning with limited use of their hands, to

specifying 'reasonable accommodations' for continuing to work."[5]

I define the "BS of MS" as an amalgam of the physical changes and

losses caused by MS, the life changes and challenges that result, and

all of the awful-feeling psychological and emotional "stuff" that comes along with those. The BS of MS comes in many forms, it runs deep, it's constant, it's really hard to wash off if it gets on you, and it can sometimes feel like quicksand. While it's not limited to just physical limitations and losses, all of it is related to those limitations and losses. Some of it launches sneak attacks or will stick a foot out and trip you; some of it will stand facing you, stare you down, and challenge you; some of it will play mind games; and, at times, all of it will pile on without heeding any notion of a "fair fight." All of it taken together can be quite heinous. It is exhausting physically, psychologically, and emotionally. At any given moment, a woman living with MS may be burdened by one or many forms of it.

The following BS of MS list is by no means comprehensive, but I feel that it covers the three major types of BS that may cause women living with MS to "live small," feel burdened, and feel defeated on a daily basis:

1. Physical Limitations BS

Women living with MS may experience physical losses, limitations, and disability. We're also likely to be experiencing some measure of grief related to those losses in addition to stress caused by uncertainty about how the disease will progress and what our level of functioning will be on any given day (we often don't know how we'll feel from morning to afternoon much less from one day to the next). While many MS-related physical limitations are visible and may have obvious ramifications to most, it's important to know that many MS-related physical limitations are not visible (for example, I suffered from debilitating MS fatigue—a very common symptom for people living with MS—for years before I had any kind of visible physical disability). And both the visible and "invisible" physical limitations are tough for us to handle psychologically and emotionally as well as physically.

For many women living with MS, the word "just" simply doesn't exist anymore for many things that require physical activity. Because of MS-related fatigue or loss of physical mobility, there may no longer be any *"Let me just get up and answer the door"* or jumping up and doing things on the fly. Seemingly simple maneuvers may be accompanied by shaky balance and a fear of the very real danger of falling. Things that we used to do quickly and on auto-pilot like simply getting dressed may now require more effort, planning, and possibly a significant amount of extra time. And the truth is that that's a very real loss that we're aware of and are reminded of every day and every time that we make a move. We may still say things out of habit that don't correspond to our current physical condition (for example, saying *"Oh, let me just run and do this"*), but be aware that our reality may be that we're experiencing significant physical limitations and losses.

2. Social Life BS

Many women living with MS may experience a disruption in their social life and relationships as a consequence of the Physical

Limitations BS mentioned above. They may feel unable to accept social invitations or participate in social activities (particularly if they are last-minute or spontaneous activities or invitations) for many reasons such as physical accessibility and/or safety concerns, fatigue, mobility issues, feeling self-conscious or awkward about their MS symptoms, self-image changes due to MS-related losses, or simply not having enough time to get ready. This can cause women living with MS to become "left out" of a social life. They may lose friends and the invitations may stop coming, eventually leading to isolation that can cause depression and make it even harder to handle MS-related challenges.

Related to this is what I like to call Socially Awkward BS. An example of this is when we're feeling down or having a rough time and friends will suggest things to us like *"Why don't you go take a walk?" [AWKWARD SILENCE]* when we can't "just" take a walk like that. We know in our hearts that they mean well and they're just forgetting because walking is not a top of mind problem for them (and neither is our particular physical condition because there's no reason for it to be), but it still hurts a bit every time we hear it. That can lead to some awkward silences or socially awkward moments. Sometimes women living with MS might avoid socializing to avoid reminders of things that they're no longer able to do or otherwise socially awkward moments, particularly if they're having a rough BS of MS day.

3. Financial BS

MS is one of the most expensive chronic diseases and it also tends to strike in the "prime of life," which often equates with prime income earning years. During these prime years and despite financial need, women living with MS often have to reduce work hours, do less-demanding work, or stop working altogether because of MS-related physical impairments. The resulting reduction in income makes it extremely difficult to handle significant current medical expenses on top of ordinary bills (not to mention the effects that it will have in the future as retirement age approaches). Because of this, at any given time, women living with MS may be experiencing serious financial stress or hardship in addition to all of the other difficulties related to MS.

The BS of MS is both physically and mentally exhausting, and it may cause women living with MS to take several hits to their self-image, self-esteem and self-confidence on top of concrete external challenges and life changes resulting from MS-related impairments. It can all feel like "too much" and lead to their feeling defeated and resigning themselves to passively living what feels like a "less than" life while the BS of MS runs the show. This book provides tools to help women overcome this BS of MS on a daily basis, so that they can lead more active and empowered-feeling lives.

MOUTH OFF ABOUT THE BS OF MS!

JOIN US FOR "BS OF MS RANT" TUESDAYS

and share what's bugging you

with other rockstar women with MS.

Get your

FREE BACKSTAGE PASS

at

www.rockstarwomenwithms.com

THREE

So, What Is This "Rockstar" Theme All About?

You'll see that I use the term "rockstar" quite often in this book. Don't worry, you don't have to sing, play an instrument or be otherwise musically-inclined; "rockstar" has nothing to do with partying or drugs; and you don't need to be a major extrovert or have a desire to be showy or flashy. I have a musical background and an affinity for the term because of my years working with bands in the independent music business, but I define the adjective "rockstar" as: The empowered and energized feeling that you get from being "in your element" and actively, consciously pursuing activities and decisions of your choice that you truly enjoy, whatever those may be for you. I created Rockstar Women With MS to help women living with MS to make rockstar decisions and live rockstar lives by making these kinds of active, conscious decisions rather than auto-pilot decisions by default or resignation simply because they have MS. My mission is to help women who are living with MS to overcome the BS of MS and create active and empowered lives that feel "rockstar" to them.

The BS of MS is a major obstacle blocking women living with MS from feeling free to live this kind of a rockstar life. Because it can create very real physical and psychological limitations that interfere with our ability to do so, the fundamental step to leading a rockstar life is learning how to overcome the BS of MS. The 3-Step Plan provided in this book will not erase the BS of MS, but it will give you the foundation tools to consistently overcome it so that you can get started on living your rockstar life.

Before we get into the Plan, I just want to say a little more about what it means, looks, or feels like to live a rockstar life or engage in a rockstar pursuit. In the "rockstar" definition above, the words "actively," "of your choice" and "whatever those may be for you" are critical here for a couple of reasons. First, doing something by settling, by default, or simply because you haven't taken the time to come up with something else that you'd like to do will not provide the same feelings of empowerment. Living life passively while letting the BS of MS control all of the decisions will cause feelings of defeat rather than empowerment, so that wouldn't feel "rockstar." Second, what someone else may consider to be a "rockstar" pursuit may not feel that way to you at all. It doesn't matter whether the rest of the world considers it to be a "rockstar" pursuit; all that matters is whether it feels that way to you.

By way of example, I'll share my own story about realizing that photography and art were NOT my "rockstar" pursuit, even though those would probably be considered by many to be an awesome thing that they'd love to be able to do. I actually struggled with the decision to leave that pursuit behind. I thought "Well, I'm good at it and I'm lucky to have the talent to do it, and it's my own personal expression, and that would be such a cool thing to do, and everyone else thinks it's such a cool thing to do, so I should want to do it (and so on, and so on) …" But, the truth is that, even as awesome as it was, it simply was not *my* "rockstar" thing. It didn't matter how "everyone else" viewed it or how many cool-points I might be able to rack up with it. What mattered was how it felt to me.

I got off of the law firm path years ago because it felt like a complete mismatch for my soul and because I wanted to work with people rather than paper. Even though it would be considered a completely opposite pursuit at first glance, I eventually realized that pursuing photography and art as a career actually felt the same as the law firm gig. Spending the majority of my time isolated in front of a computer screen felt like the equivalent of that super-limited "just working with paper" feeling I'd had at the firm, even though creating art is something that I actually love to do. When I really looked deep inside, I saw that I lacked a fire in my gut to pursue it as more than just a side project. It wasn't truly my passion, and isolation for 70% of the time wasn't a match for my personality (I'm an off-the-charts "extrovert" according to Myers-Briggs testing). I came to realize that the work I'd been doing helping to build a nonprofit organization serving other women with MS is what felt more aligned with a real "rockstar" match for me. That led me down my eventual path to discovering that coaching and helping to guide other women with MS along their own rockstar journeys was MY "rockstar" pursuit, while creating art was best enjoyed in a part-time or hobby status.

Before you delve into the 3-Step Plan, I'd like you to consider what you feel that a "rockstar" life would look like for you. What would your "rockstar" activity or pursuit be? What makes you feel empowered, energized and truly "in your element?" Have you been afraid to pursue it because you have MS? If you could successfully learn to overcome the BS of MS, would you pursue it? What kinds of "rockstar" decisions would you love to make?

COME SHARE YOUR "ROCKSTAR" VISION!

Come share your "rockstar" activities and vision with us.

If you don't know what those are yet,

we can support you in finding them.

Get your

FREE BACKSTAGE PASS

at

www.rockstarwomenwithms.com

FOUR

3-STEP PLAN Step One: Building Your Must-Have-Rockstar-Toolkit
(The 10 Tools That You MUST Have In Your Arsenal)

Okay, here is where it gets good. The 3-Step Plan that's spelled out in these next 3 chapters is a system of preparation, personal empowerment, and conscious forward action that is designed to help women living with MS to consistently overcome the BS of MS. It gives you the tools to get a grip on it, manage it like a boss, prevail over it, and start racking up wins so that you can feel enabled to actively create a life that feels rockstar to you. And the great thing is that you can start implementing the Plan right away.

I'm sure the first question that's been looming in your mind has got to be "How and where do I even *begin* to deal with this BS of MS?"

Well, you start here with Step One: Assembling your Must-Have-Rockstar-Toolkit. This Toolkit is what's going to give you a solid foundation to start overcoming the BS of MS so that you can start creating the life that you want to live. It will help you to build and maintain confidence, create and keep the headspace that you'll need to keep moving forward toward your goals, and help to act as a bumper when you run up against any physical or mental bumps and bruises along the way. This chapter will lay out these must-have tools for you in detail and point you to some ways to start building your own personal Toolkit right away.

In order to begin and then to persist in living a rockstar life while living with the BS of MS, you must have an array of resources available to motivate and support you. Some of these resources will be internal, some will be external, and there are many that you will have to build and tweak as you go. You may feel impatient to move forward or tempted to procrastinate on this, but you really must start building this Toolkit as your first step. Once you've started getting these tools in place, you can really move forward in creating your rockstar life; but, if you skip this step, you will get or remain stuck. Or you will start to make a little progress and then have a major backslide pretty quickly. I can almost guarantee it (trust me on this one). So, really commit to putting your Toolkit in place as your first step, okay?

So, here are the 10 powerful tools that you need to have in your arsenal to support you in your rockstar journey to consistently overcome the BS of MS:

Rockstar Tool #1: A Rocket-Powered Motivation

I would have been perfectly happy never having learned to knit. *"Oh, you can make yourself a sweater"* held no motivation whatsoever for me and still doesn't. I didn't and don't need to make myself a sweater, and I was and still am pretty sure that I don't want a sweater that looks like I made it, anyway. Being a non-knitter wouldn't have bothered me one bit…

Until the day that I heard the story of a child with AIDS in Africa who had been given a hand-knit teddy bear and said he wanted to be buried with it because it was his only friend (*Good Lord, can you feel my heart breaking right now???*). From that moment on, I would have moved heaven and earth to learn how to knit teddy bears just to make sure that I could get "friends" to children like that. I didn't care whether I never learned how to knit anything else but bears, but I was going to learn how to do that if it was the last thing I did in this lifetime. A dear friend taught me and I learned to knit bears in a couple of weeks, and my bears continue to provide comfort to sick and underprivileged children worldwide. I still haven't knitted a sweater and I probably never will.

I also said that I'd NEVER write a book because, even though I've always loved writing, I just didn't have the attention span for it. But, guess what? Wanting to write this book for you and to help women living with MS like myself blew that never writing a book thing off the road.

Funny how that works, right?

I share these stories to make the point that our motivation determines and propels the choices that we make in life, including whether we decide to take a backseat to the BS of our MS or decide to choose otherwise. And defeating inertia or truly changing the path that you're currently on requires a motivation that's the right one for YOU...an inspiring motivation that you just can't say no to, even if you'd like to. Creating a rockstar life while living with MS requires an inspiration or motivation of equally rockstar proportions, and it has to feel like it's of rockstar proportions to *you personally*. It doesn't matter what it feels like to someone else. Their motivation may not be a match for you and may not be enough to get you moving.

So, what's *your* motivation for wanting to overcome the BS of MS and make changes in your life? Are you fed-up with feeling like the BS of MS makes or drives most (*All?*) of your life decisions? Are you sick of feeling like a wallflower or like you're living life on the sidelines? Are you desperate to get off of the bench and get into the game to show family and friends (*Or even yourself?*) what you're truly made of? What's your greatest and deepest motivation? THAT'S the one that you need to connect with and channel in order to pursue your rockstar life transformation. Really dig deep and think about this. Find that motivation and you've found the equivalent of rocket fuel.

You can read about others' motivations and share your own in our community of rockstar women with MS by picking up your free Backstage Pass at rockstarwomenwithms.com.

Rockstar Tool #2: A Clear Vision

A clear vision will help you to focus and recharge your rocket-powered motivation as well as keep you from burning up your time and energy flailing around without a plan. Create your vision of what your "rockstar" life looks like. As we discussed above, don't worry about what a "rockstar" life looks like for other people or what society and the media tell you that it "should" look like—What is YOUR vision for who you want to be, how you want to feel, and what you want to create in your life?

Have fun with this, really dream big, and really see and feel yourself in your vision as if it already exists. Don't worry yet about the HOW of it all. The secret is that you don't need to know the HOW first. Create a vision section in your journal, make a physical vision board, or make a virtual one on your computer. Write about your vision and add pictures, article clippings, quotes, etc., to really immerse and feel yourself in it.

Once you know what your vision is, you will be bolstered in taking concrete action steps to help you to achieve it.

Grab your free Backstage Pass at rockstarwomenwithms.com to share your vision and find support in achieving it.

Rockstar Tool #3: A Belief In Options

The third tool that you need to have in your arsenal is a belief that you:

1) Have options (even if you can't see them at that very moment), and

2) Have the ability to create additional options for yourself most of the time. It is important to understand and respect the realities of Multiple Sclerosis in order to keep yourself physically safe. That being said, you also need to be aware of what kinds of limiting beliefs or self-talk may be holding you back without a foundation in medical reality.

I listened to my doctor, but chose to believe in and create options for myself. I knew that it was important to understand and be respectful of the medical and physical facts about my condition; but I also knew that no two cases of MS were the same, I knew how my own body felt and responded, and I chose to believe that I had more options than the standard fare of stuff that we hear would lead me to believe. That allowed me to have a mindset from which I could actively pursue and create lifestyle options for myself.

Now, I don't at all intend to imply that this was easy for me because it was not. In fact, building this Belief In Options tool was one of the hardest things that I've ever done because, at that particular time in my life, I was pretty much starting the build from scratch. I had a string of events happen that left me really feeling beaten-down to the point where I felt that I was at the bottom of a well where I couldn't even see a speck of light at the top. That feeling of being so deep in it that I didn't know how far away the top was (if there even was a top) was awful because it felt like there might be no point in even trying to start climbing out. Besides, I didn't even trust that I'd have the strength or ability to do it. Let me tell you, that period of time was one of the worst things that I'd ever experienced. My confidence was shot, my belief in my abilities had taken a huge hit, and my belief in the options available to me had not just been limited, but had been decimated.

So, I had to start building a new Belief In Options…and I used a series of tools to rebuild that belief brick-by-brick until I felt ready to start trying to climb out of the well. And I eventually got myself out.

Limiting beliefs are going to be the major gremlins interfering with your building your Belief In Options tool. The truth is that limiting beliefs are a huge topic and it would probably require writing at least one whole book to discuss them. As I'm sure that there are many people who have already done just that in a splendid manner and there are tons of good books available for you to learn more about them, I will simply say this: Limiting beliefs are very real and very powerful, and I'd bet money that you have some. We all have them.

So, what beliefs do you currently have about the options that are available to you? What are the thoughts and self-talk that have been circulating in your head for the past several months?   How about yesterday? Today?

To learn more about limiting beliefs and get help with effectively busting the beliefs that may be holding you back, pick up your free Backstage Pass and discover new resources at rockstarwomenwithms.com.

Rockstar Tool #4: A Sense Of Humor (You HAVE To Laugh)

You know, you just have to be able to see the humor in things. Especially on this particular journey with the BS of MS (What do they say? "You have to laugh to keep from crying?"). C'mon, you have to admit that you can see the humor in this sometimes. Not in terms of funny, ha-ha, but in terms of absurdity on occasion. You know, at those times when it seems like it's some colossal joke that there are now new "rules" that make things harder or more absurd just because you have MS. For example, the new rule that if you drop something, it will not just fall but will roll far away and more likely than not end up underneath something just because it's now 18 times harder for you to stand up, then bend down and get something, much less crawl under some furniture to do it and get back up. Or how it's not possible to laugh and walk at the same time. Or when you go out with your MS girlfriends and you all share a huge belly laugh at the moment you all simultaneously throw your purses on the floor before standing up because none of you can get up while holding them, and you realize that you're all using this same technique.

I've gotten tangled in a Christmas tree (in public) and had to be rescued because my cane got caught, I've had senior citizens offer me their walker seats and offer to carry my groceries on many occasions (and I've said no when I really wanted to say yes because they walked better than I did), and seniors always blow right by me on the street because they move much faster than I do. And that's just the tip of the iceberg of my stockpile of MS situations that are simply ridiculous. And embarrassing. And feel just awful. And yet I have laughed to the point of tears over many of these things because they're funny— Couldn't help myself because the absurdity of them was humorous. And I've learned that this kind of stuff creates immediate bonds with other women who also have MS, whether they are already friends of mine or we have just met…because they "get" it (after all, we already share some inside jokes before we've even met).

And being able to see the humor in some of this absurdity is also what can save you when you're feeling at your lowest points. Right after I had accomplished a milestone cane-less walk around my block (which I hadn't been able to do for a year), I came into my apartment and fell not even 10 minutes after I got home. I definitely was not seeing the humor in that at the time…it felt more like a defeat or a cruel joke having what should have been a moment of triumph snatched right out from under me before I'd even had time to enjoy it. My immediate reaction was a combination of fear, wondering whether I was hurt, sadness, and a quick flash of *"Am I kidding myself by being on this great mission that I have?"* But, in an instant, that was all wiped out by the thought *"Ooh! There's my extension cord!!"* Lying on the floor where I was, I found myself at direct eye-level with the extension cord that I'd been looking for for days curled up beneath my couch. Couldn't help laughing. Loudly. Sometimes, that's all it takes to keep going. And that's why a sense of humor is a must-have tool in your arsenal.

Bond and have a laugh with a great community of other rockstar women with MS who "get" it by sharing your humorous/absurd MS moments or personal take on the new "rules." Get your free Backstage Pass at rockstarwomenwithms.com.

Rockstar Tool #5: Proper Nutrition and Exercise

If you don't take care of your body, you simply don't have your full capacity to do anything, whether you have a medical condition or not. I was honest with myself that, even though I was (mostly) following my medication regimen, I was not truly doing what was required to keep my body healthy overall.

I had done a lot of research on nutrition and eating regimens that were beneficial for people with MS, I'd learned about what supplements could also help, and I already knew full-well about the benefits of doing some kind of regular exercise. But, knowing and doing are two very different things—The problem was that knowing these things didn't help me if I wasn't implementing them. The reality was that I weighed a little too much, didn't follow a good nutrition regimen consistently, and wasn't doing anywhere near what could be considered "regular" exercise (other than flexing my "justification muscles" with the built-in excuse of a persistent ankle injury, even though that totally didn't fly for several exercises that I could have been doing). And the results of that showed in my fatigue levels, my decreasing mobility, and how I felt in general. No good at all. I knew that I had to change that.

And further incentive to get myself moving came when I learned that the old advice about exercise not being good for people living with MS is rapidly being debunked. In fact, physical therapy and exercise are increasingly being shown to be helpful in modifying mobility loss for people living with MS. Dr. Herb Karpatkin, an assistant professor of physical therapy at Hunter College in New York confirms this, stating:

> "Exercise must be an essential part of treatment for anyone with Multiple Sclerosis. It is as important as medication. The reason for this is that Multiple Sclerosis is a disease of mobility. While MD's may be looking at the effects of MS

on myelin, what you as a patient notice is that MS slowly takes away your ability to walk, balance, and move the way that you want to. While medication may slow the course of the disease, it does little if anything to restore lost mobility. The only way to improve mobility is to practice mobility. Difficulties with walking can best be improved by practicing walking. Difficulties with balance are best improved by practicing balance. Unfortunately the opposite is also true; difficulty with walking often leads persons with MS to walk less, and this results in walking ability decreasing further. Difficulties with balance often lead persons with MS to avoid situations that lead to balance loss, and this leads to a progressive avoidance of postures and movements that challenge balance at all, leaving the person more and more sedentary. Being sedentary is a major reason for morbidity and mortality in persons with MS. This will happen regardless of the effectiveness of disease modifying medication.

On the other hand, numerous studies have shown the effectiveness of exercise in modifying the mobility loss associated with MS. In fact, it may be that a significant portion of the disability seen in MS is not due to the disease itself but due to the sedentary lifestyle that far too many persons with MS seem to adopt. This is actually very good news for persons with MS, as it suggests that a large portion of their disability may in fact be reversible through something that is free, safe, and easily accessible: Exercise."

I began eating according to recommended nutrition, and I began physical exercise regimens (even though it was psychologically and physically hard for me as a former athlete to basically be starting from zero in the fitness department, I knew that I had to start somewhere).

Even though I still haven't yet returned to being "in shape" like I used to be, I'm working on it, and I can tell you firsthand that making the conscious efforts that I have to prioritize my physical health has made a world of difference.   A stronger and healthier body—and even seeing that it's possible to improve my strength, stability, and mobility in the first place—has made me feel a greater sense of positivity and possibility overall.   It will also do the same for you.   So, do your research on improving your nutrition, speak with your doctor about physical therapy and exercise, and prioritize incorporating all of these safely and consistently into your regular routine.

I can tell you from my own personal experience that: 1) It's a lot easier to manage the BS of MS in general if you're not feeling physically lousy due to poor nutrition, and 2) Some of the Physical Limitations BS may actually lessen when you make a conscious effort to do some kind of regular exercise or physical therapy.

Rockstar Tool #6: An Ability To Create Your Own Support Tools

Even if we're fortunate to have stellar support from family, friends and a medical team, there are still going to be times when they will be unavailable or just not capable of giving us the type of support that we need.   At times, because of their care and concern, they may unwittingly discourage us and keep our thinking limited.   There will also be times when we feel that it's not appropriate or will not be supportive to turn to them. In instances like these, we need to have our own personal support tools at-the-ready.   I developed my own set of tools to build and bolster my confidence and persistence in order to support myself in those instances when outside support might not be available, and you can do that, too.

You're going to need two sets of personalized support tools. You will need to have heavy-duty support tools that will do the heavy lifting for you in the background on an ongoing basis, and you'll also need a set of simple tools at-the-ready to quickly support yourself on-the-spot when you need to. The heavy-duty tools require some time to build because of the work you'll need to do to customize them effectively for yourself (you can find in-depth help for doing that at rockstarwomenwithms.com); so we'll focus here on the simple tools that you can start putting in place while you build the heavy lifters.

The job of your simple support tools is to change or clear your energy state quickly. You may already have a couple of these tools that you've been using to support yourself all along. Think about it...what tools do you already use or have at-the-ready to support yourself when things get tough? These "tools" would be things that you already know help you to flip-switch out of a negative state, to feel energized, or to reduce your stress level.

In order to switch off a negative state and get a power boost when I start to feel discouraged, I have a few Go-To tools that always work. The tool that works first and foremost for me is music because I absolutely love it, and the right music will switch me into an empowered state pretty much immediately. For me, Soundgarden is my go-to when I really need to feel empowered from my core. It's one of my favorite bands, their music has always somehow connected with and energized me at a core level, and I associate their music with the soundtrack from some of the most powerful times in my life. I also channel my inner Led Zeppelin. I've got an iconic picture of them from back in the day hanging above my desk (right next to a picture of my Dad that makes me feel supported every time that I look at it). There's no way that you can see or think about Robert Plant in all fabulousness on stage and not feel inspired to switch into some kind of rockstar state yourself.

Music is just one example of the many simple personal support tools that I have in my arsenal (knitting teddy bears is another one). I have simple support tools like these in addition to the heavy-duty customized tools that I've created to consistently do the heavy lifting in the background for me on a daily basis. And I know that I have the ability to create additional tools or tweak the ones that no longer seem to be working as well for me.

While you're learning to create your own heavy-duty support tools, get started on finding what works for you as a simple personal support tool to help switch you out of a negative state. It may not be music… maybe it's yoga, meditation, drawing, gardening, or something else. The point is to use whatever makes you feel amazing and can really flip-switch you into either a more peaceful or a more powerful energy state.

IMPORTANT CAVEAT: If you have gotten into the habit of emotional overeating, an eating disorder, or any kind of substance abuse as a mood-adjuster or coping mechanism, that does NOT qualify as a "rockstar" support tool. That will do you more harm than good, and will directly neutralize the benefits of the very important Rockstar

Tool #5.

Rockstar Tool #7: External Support Resources

Ideally, you will have external support from family and friends as well

as your medical team.   If you don't, there are several resources

available to help you find external support; and, even if you do already

have support, it's a good idea to further bolster your support arsenal by

availing yourself of these options as well.

Nonprofit organizations like the National Multiple Sclerosis Society

(www.nationalmssociety.org) are a wonderful source of support and

can provide you with information about support groups, psychologists

and social workers, and an extensive range of programs, services,

resources and connection opportunities.   Doing some online research

can help you find organizations like this as well as support services in

your local area; and, thanks to the Internet and our increasingly

connected world, there are opportunities for you to participate in support services via telephone or online mechanisms as well as in person.

Also, definitely reach out to and connect with other women living with MS because they can understand and support you in what you're going through in a way that people without MS just cannot. And they "get" it on more than just the level of experiencing similar physical symptoms or losses. They "get" the humor that we talked about earlier, they "get" the loss you feel in no longer being able to wear cute shoes and somehow feeling less feminine, and they "get" your envy of people who can wear flip-flops or who can walk while simultaneously carrying a coffee and talking on a cell phone without fear of tripping and falling. They understand why these things that may seem trivial to or go unnoticed by others actually mean a lot.

And, by the way, you're going to find out that you've also got cheerleaders that you don't even know about who will contribute to

building the energy in your external support network. It was beyond
cool for me to learn that people are on the sidelines rooting for me that
I didn't even know existed. Even though I know that we humans (a lot
of us, anyway) have it in us to root for the underdog and to want to see
people succeed (After all, isn't that why we'll line marathon routes to
cheer people on that we don't even know?), I didn't expect to have my
own cheering section; but, I have now had several of then crop up in
different places.

There are a couple of supporters in my neighborhood that I now know
about, whom I've chatted with on the street and who have encouraged
me to keep up my walking practice; but one day I was really surprised
to meet a cheerleader that I didn't even know existed. When I was out
practicing walking one morning, a man came out of a building to give
me well wishes and see how I was doing. I told him that I'd lost some
ground because of the weather the past winter, but was getting back
out there and doing better than before. And he said *"I know."*

Apparently, he's seen the efforts I've made at this walking thing in the past year or two, and he's aware of my progress. I remember when it was a struggle for me to get to the corner and back. Maybe he remembers that, too? Anyway, he encouraged me, and said he'd seen my progress and was thinking to himself *"Look at that pretty lady go!"* He told me to let him know if I ever need any help. Wow.

Learning that I've actually got silent support out there that I didn't know about from people that I don't even know was a real eye-opener. It keeps me motivated and also helps me to feel buoyed by a "cloud" of good energy.

Visit rockstarwomenwithms.com to bond with and find external support in a great community of other rockstar women with MS.

Rockstar Tool #8: Make Yourself Feel Beautiful

This is something that may seem superficial at first glance, but this is truly not just about vanity and should be taken seriously for several reasons (you'll see...I've even got citations coming up in a moment).

We women face constant societal pressures and stereotypes concerning

our appearance, regardless of whether we have an illness or disability;

[6] and how we feel about our appearance directly correlates with our

self-esteem. How a woman feels about how she looks can

unfortunately make or break her self-esteem or what she believes is

possible for her. It's been shown that increased self-esteem actually

magnifies our perception of available resources and their

effectiveness[7] as well as our own ability to cope with and adapt to the

daily challenges of MS.[8]

So, how we feel about our appearance goes beyond the general "when

you look good, you feel good" thing that we've probably all heard

before. When a woman with MS feels good about her appearance, her

perception of her own abilities and possibilities—in other words, her

Belief In Options (BAM!—Rockstar Tool #3!) improves.

While helping women through my nonprofit organization, I witnessed

firsthand the consistent positive transformations in energy and attitude

experienced by women with MS who received makeovers and felt

empowered by learning adapted personal grooming and makeup

application techniques.   And I've found that making even simple

efforts with my own appearance (like even just wearing my signature

red lipstick) boosted my self-esteem and perceptions of my abilities to

actively improve my life.

So, yes, how you feel about your appearance matters.   Make yourself

feel beautiful.

Join us at rockstarwomenwithms.com to see upcoming events about

adaptive grooming and makeup application techniques, and to share

your own feelings and tips concerning appearance and beauty

regimens.

Rockstar Tool #9: Exercise Your Gratitude & Helping-Others Muscles

When you're feeling low, it's hard to maintain perspective, and it's very easy to fall into a limited and negative headspace. At my lowest point when I was desperate to snap myself out of having felt lousy for so long, I knew that one way to have a more positive mindset would be to start being actively and consciously mindful of and grateful for what I had. And I knew that the second thing that I had to do was take the focus off of myself and start to help others. I began a gratitude journal, I helped to build a nonprofit organization that helps other women living with MS, I became an active volunteer in the MS community, and I began knitting teddy bears for sick and underprivileged children. After a while, my change of focus to gratitude and helping others became natural rather than something that required conscious effort, and exercising these "muscles" consistently helps me to keep my mind more open and positive.

You can start exercising your gratitude muscles right away in many different ways. Starting a gratitude journal is an easy way to start. Another great way to exercise and project your gratitude is to simply start owning and rocking what you've got on a daily basis. I may need a cane to walk right now, but I'm grateful to have that cane as a tool to help me get around and I proudly dress it up and rock it when I go out. I've got cheetah-print, zebra-print, and sparkly cane covers for it that fit my style and make the cane feel and look more like a positive fashion accessory than a dreary-feeling medical aid. And the cane covers also give other people a smile and a boost of positive energy when they see them (and kids just love the sparkly cover...I've seen them keep turning around to look at it even after they've gotten halfway down the block).

So, what are you grateful for, and how can you start consciously exercising that gratitude? What are some ways in which you could use your talents to help others or support a good cause?

Rockstar Tool #10: Mobility Aids And Transportation Assistance

Okay, this is a tough one for a lot of us. It certainly was a tough one for me. Mobility aids such as canes, walkers, and wheelchairs; and transportation assistance through paratransit programs actually are rockstar tools, even though they may not psychologically or emotionally feel like that for many of us. They may painfully represent and remind us of physical losses experienced because of MS, and we may put up a lot of resistance to using them because we fear losing more mobility/ability and because we don't want to feel like we're "disabled" yet or be identified as "disabled." But the truth of the matter is that not using these aids and forms of transportation assistance when they're available to us is not a rockstar move. Don't kid yourself—You do NOT get any bonus cool-points for endangering your physical safety or for being and feeling physically wiped-out when you had a different option available.

I understand how hard it is to experience continuing physical losses from MS and to start realizing the need for mobility assistance. I remember how it felt to go from having a cane folded up in my bag 90% of the time to needing to use it 100% of the time, and I remember when I first started to need wheelchair assistance in airports and train stations. I struggled with the thought of getting transportation assistance through the paratransit services that are available where I live. I figured *"Well, if I can still walk around even though it's a struggle and I'm hobbling with a cane and I don't feel that safe and it will take forever, I'm still walking...I can still make it...I'm not 'disabled' yet..."* I struggled on like that for a couple of years before finally taking advantage of the paratransit services that were offered to me, and what a positive difference that has made in my life! I wish that I had started using those services earlier, but the truth is simply that I wasn't psychologically or emotionally ready yet. Let me save you some of the time, energy, money, and opportunities that I lost by not doing it sooner.

The amount of time, physical energy, and access that we lose by not taking advantage of the transportation services and mobility devices available to us is extraordinary. These types of options allow us to have rockstar lives because they allow us to travel, help us to conserve our physical strength and energy, and help us to have more time to put to positive use (because it's not spent struggling to get around or recovering from the struggle to get around). They allow us to have more mobility and ability than we would have without them. Speak to your doctor or physical therapist about mobility devices that might help you, and research the paratransit services that are available in your local area. Several railway companies and airlines offer wheelchair services, so you can also travel out of town safely. These are all tools that are definitely rockstar tools, and my advice to you is to take advantage of them and have them in your toolkit. They will increase the number of options that you're going to have available to you as you work on creating your rockstar life experiences.

NEED HELP BUILDING YOUR TOOLKIT?

For resources, guidance, and

community support to help you

build your Must-Have-Rockstar-Toolkit,

visit

www.rockstarwomenwithms.com

FIVE

3-STEP PLAN Step Two:
Begin Cultivating Your Rockstar Mindset

Now that you've successfully completed the first step of building your Must-Have-Rockstar-Toolkit, you're ready for the second step, which is to begin cultivating a rockstar mindset. You are truly going to need this mindset in order to consistently overcome the BS of MS.

Your thoughts are where your real power lies—Your mindset can make you or break you. Unfortunately, you can't think your way out of crappy thoughts more often than not, so what you have to do is make sure that you improve the overall quality of your thoughts to begin with. So, how do you do that? The truth is that doing that effectively is a long-term and ongoing process that's beyond the scope of this chapter (and even beyond the scope of this handbook). Programs and resources are available to give you long-term help with this at rockstarwomenwithms.com, but what I'm going to do right now is give you some kickstart fundamentals so that you can begin cultivating your rockstar mindset.

Rockstar Mindset Kickstart Fundamental #1: 3 Questions

In order to start building a rockstar mindset, you must first get a handle on what your headspace looks like right now (You can't get to your destination if you don't know where you're starting on the map, right?), and I'm going to ask you three questions about this. My first question to you is this: What is it that you believe about yourself with your condition that currently holds you back? Notice that I didn't ask you what it is about MS, but what it is that you believe about *yourself* with MS that currently holds you back. I know that may sound a little confusing, but what I mean by that is: How do you see yourself with MS in terms of what your own personal abilities are to live a life that you would like to live? I ask that because there are many people who also have MS that are doing amazing things. Do you think that there's something you personally lack that prevents you from doing amazing things, too?

Really think about this first question. It's going to be one key to uncovering the reasons why you may be on a path in your life right now that you don't like or the reasons that you may have gotten stuck, and it also directly relates to your Rockstar Tool #3 Belief In Options. Do you currently have a belief in options, or do you see your options as severely limited? You have to know the answer to that first; and, if you see your options as severely limited, then that's something that you will have to change in order to successfully overcome the BS of MS. Please realize that you are not your MS. You are not your disability. The MS and any disability that you may be experiencing are challenges that you have, they are not who you are. Even changing your perception of how you identify yourself with the illness will change your perception of what options you have available to you.

My second question to you is this: Were any of these beliefs that you just thought about the same *before* you had MS? Be truly honest with yourself as to what you believed was possible for you and what options were available to you *before* you had MS. I ask you this because you have to have an awareness of any limiting beliefs that you're starting with right now that are unrelated to the MS itself. You may have some long-held limiting beliefs hanging around that were with you long before you were diagnosed with MS.

The third question to ask yourself is how good you're willing to have your life be. You may be thinking *"Huh?? I want my life to be great... what are you talking about?"* But, is that really 100% true? You may never have thought about this before, but you probably have subconsciously or even consciously identified and labeled yourself in terms of what you're "allowed" to have or what you deserve in life. Those are the thoughts that sound like *"I'm not one of those people who gets to [fill in the blank]"* or *"I could never [fill in the blank]."*

The truth of the matter is that you may have an "upper limit problem" that will cause you to sabotage your efforts to make rockstar changes in your life, so you need to find out if that's the case.

Gay Hendricks has actually written a great book about this upper limit problem called *The Big Leap.*[9] If you're having an upper limit problem, you may be unconsciously sabotaging yourself because you actually can only tolerate your life being a certain level of "good." How comfortable do you feel with experiencing joy or success? When something amazingly great happens to you, do you immediately start wondering what's going to go wrong or start waiting for the proverbial "other shoe" to drop? Do you often steal your moments of joy or success out from under yourself like that right away because you feel on some level that you personally don't get to have things like that in your life, or that you somehow don't deserve it? Perhaps someone in your past discouraged you and warned you against playing too large, standing out, having high expectations, or "getting your hopes up?" Or perhaps you had an experience (or more than one) of trying to break out of your habit of lying low and you got shot down, and then decided consciously or subconsciously to never let that happen again...either to protect yourself or because you simply identified yourself as "not one of those people who gets to have/do/be" whatever that thing is. All of these things contribute to and indicate the upper limit that you are currently willing and able to tolerate.

We spoke earlier about having to exercise certain "muscles" like your gratitude muscles and your literal physical muscles, but you're also going to have to do some mental stretching and strengthening to raise the upper limit that you're able to tolerate. Really ask yourself how much success, happiness, joy, and putting yourself out there you're really comfortable with. Be honest with yourself: If you didn't have MS, would reaching for any of your dreams make you feel too uncomfortable for you to even try? When you imagine yourself achieving those dreams or when you picture yourself in your vision of your ideal life, do you feel uncomfortable? If you feel a knot in your chest or stomach (or even feel yourself wanting to snicker), that indicates discomfort on some level and is a clue as to what you're currently able to tolerate. The MS is certainly a legitimate reason for not doing certain things; but it can also be a good excuse or "red herring" in many situations that distracts from the reality that we may also have an upper limit problem that has nothing to do with the MS.

If you find that you're really struggling with limited thinking or an upper limit problem, then you may need some extra assistance with busting some heavy-duty limiting beliefs. As I mentioned earlier, the topic of limiting beliefs is too enormous to cover thoroughly in this handbook, and working through your own may take a while (fear not, though, there are several programs and resources available to help you with that when you're ready at rockstarwomenwithms.com). The step that I want you to take right now, though, is simply to recognize what your mindset happens to be at this moment...what your level of belief in options for yourself with MS happens to be right now. Know that you may have to change it, and if you feel that you do have to change it, then commit to doing the future work to do so. Even just the step of making that commitment to yourself will already start to create a rockstar mindset in you.

Rockstar Mindset Kickstart Fundamental #2: Feel Your Feelings

The second necessary piece for cultivating your rockstar mindset is giving yourself the space and permission to feel your feelings about MS. You absolutely must feel your feelings regarding having MS and any disability that you may be experiencing. We can't kick-start you into action that you can sustain if you're trying to hide, ignore, or bury those feelings. That would be a setup for a backslide because these feelings will undermine your mindset and ultimately come back to sabotage you somewhere in your rockstar journey or somewhere else in your life.

I know that it may be painful to pull up and acknowledge these feelings. I also understand that trying to hide, ignore, or bury them may be a coping mechanism that you have been using to help you get through interactions with other people or to even just get through your day; but, part of your healthy rockstar mindset will be accepting and allowing yourself to feel the feelings that you have about your MS and your disability because they're valid. Allowing yourself to feel them is empowering because you'll see that you can give that to yourself without falling apart, and you will also have a conscious awareness of them that will prevent them from sneaking up to sabotage you later.

Rockstar Mindset Kickstart Fundamental #3

And, last but not least, the third part of cultivating your rockstar mindset is to build the right set of tools that will bolster, shield, and bulletproof your new rockstar thinking and beliefs about yourself (think of it like a maintenance program to keep pests away, so that they won't damage your growing crops). That is a long-term project that needs to be customized for you to truly be effective, so it's also something that can't be done overnight; but we can help you build these tools at rockstarwomenwithms.com. The kick-start step that you can take right now is simply to commit to giving yourself that gift in the future.

BUST
THOSE
BELIEFS!

To get help with discovering

and busting your limiting beliefs

or help cultivating your rockstar mindset,

visit

www.rockstarwomenwithms.com

SIX

3-STEP PLAN Step Three: Start Setting And Acting On Some "Impossible" Goals

This may seem like the scariest step, but it also ends up being the most rewarding and the biggest confidence-builder. The third step in overcoming the BS of MS is to start setting some "impossible" goals for yourself and then begin acting on them. This step will help to reinforce your new rockstar mindset and expand your Belief In Options (Rockstar Tool #3). This is also where you will really begin to see and feel some forward progress in creating a new life for yourself that is not dictated by the BS of MS.

By "impossible" goals, I don't mean dangerous goals that in any way threaten your health, safety, or well-being; and I don't mean goals that are patently unrealistic (you can't be a doctor if you haven't gone to medical school). By "impossible," I mean something that, in the way that you've been thinking or feeling recently, you believe is simply out of your league or beyond your reach. And you know that we all exaggerate and label those things as "impossible," even though that may not be factually true. THOSE are the kinds of goals that I want you to start setting for yourself.

Back in Chapter 5, we discussed limiting beliefs that sound and feel like *"I'm not one of those people who gets to [fill in the blank]"* or *"I could never [fill in the blank]."* What are some things that you would really like to do, be, or have? When you think of them, does your mind automatically default to a limiting belief that sounds or feels like that? If that's the case, then I want you to pick one of those things as a goal and start taking action to achieve it.

If you just gasped or froze up, don't panic.

You may be thinking that this is easier said than done…and you're right. But, you CAN do it.

Start small. It doesn't have to be an enormous or complicated goal, and you don't have to take the biggest, scariest step first. You don't have to start where you ultimately plan to end up or anywhere even close to that. Don't overwhelm yourself in your own mind. Even if you don't know exactly how to achieve your first "impossible" goal yet, you will figure it out.

Do your research and find out what it will take to achieve the first "impossible" goal that you want to achieve, outline an overall plan, and then write down the first action steps that you need to take to get started. Then start taking action. The truth is that you've actually already taken two steps by doing your research and then writing down those action steps (Yes, I tricked you into taking action already and you didn't even know it, so you've already started!), so taking the first action step that you wrote down is really already your third step! You take that step. And then you take the next step. If you find that you're going to need to do more research to find out what the next steps toward achieving your goal should be, then you repeat the process: Do that next round of research, write down the next set of action steps that you'll need to take, and act on those steps, too.

Continue this pattern to inch your way along the path to your ultimate goal. If you really catch on to it quickly and decide that you're ready and want to move by leaps and bounds, then by all means, go ahead and do that. But, if you're not ready for that or not comfortable with that yet, then move baby step by baby step and inch your way along. The main point here is that you continue taking conscious forward action. By taking this action, you'll build up your confidence and, before you know it, you'll reach your first "impossible" goal. And then you'll be ready to start tackling your next "impossible" goal.

Continue taking action on the "impossible" goals that you've set, achieve those, and then set some more. As you rack up achievements and see yourself achieve goal after goal, then both your confidence and your Belief In Options will grow tremendously. You will also see yourself starting to have the upper hand in overcoming the BS of MS as you begin seeing that you are exerting more conscious control over your time and how you choose to use it in addition to learning what you are truly capable of doing with it.

A HELPFUL TIP IF YOU FIND YOURSELF FREEZING UP ON THIS STEP: You may find yourself freezing up even at the thought of picking out a goal much less making an attempt to achieve it. Why is that? It could be that you have a major limiting belief or upper limit problem hanging you up, or it could be that you are stuck because you're a perfectionist and you don't feel "ready" or "good enough" to act yet. If your problem is the former, then you may need some extra help to get you started (and you can visit rockstarwomenwithms.com to get help with that); and, if your problem is the latter, then acting "as if" can help to get you unstuck.

You may have heard of the advice to act "as if" before. It basically means to act "as if" we have achieved or manifested something that we want to (even if we haven't yet), that something we want is happening for us (even if it's not yet), or that we are "good enough" to achieve what we want (even if we don't feel like it yet). Well, that's actually good advice, and that's what I suggest that you do because it's a good way to get you to start taking any action at all.

What I know from personal experience is that, if you wait until you feel like you're "ready" or "good enough" to take action towards achieving a goal, then you will wait for a long time (as a recovering perfectionist, that's what I used to do). And then you will wait some more. Procrastination makes a great bedfellow for people who are perpetually "getting ready to get ready," so don't be one of those people.   Act "as if" in order to get yourself moving on those action steps toward your "impossible" goal, even if you don't fully believe in yourself yet and are freaking out on the inside (Keep your cool and no one will know that but you!). As you act "as if," believe that you can achieve your goal and be the new vision that you have for yourself (And, if you find yourself hesitating, think of it this way: If your odds of pulling it off are an even 50/50 for "yes" or "no," then why not choose to believe "YES" because that will make you feel good and help you to take action?).

Once you've become a pro at acting "as if," you'll find yourself naturally continuing to take action without feeling like an impostor. There's no need for you to feel like an impostor because you've already built a track record of successfully achieving by taking action!

GET READY, ALREADY!

Take that first step and

connect with our

free support community at

ROCKSTAR WOMEN WITH MS.

Get your

FREE BACKSTAGE PASS

at
www.rockstarwomenwithms.com

SEVEN

The Inevitable BS of MS—What To Do If You Get Stuck

Even though we have now begun cultivating a rockstar mindset and started making forward progress on achieving "impossible" goals, it would be irresponsible for me to let you think that it will all be smooth sailing from hereon in. Because it won't be. The Harsh Reality is that, as we move forward on our rockstar journeys, we're going to continue facing the BS of MS daily (unfortunately, it doesn't just disappear)... we may slow down, get fatigued, experience vision problems, stumble and fall, and lose functionalities that we've taken for granted that we may or may not get back—And there is no denying that these are very real obstacles (and they are challenges that we will have to face IN ADDITION to all of the regular drama that shows up in everyone's lives, anyway). BUT, the Rockstar Reality is this: Our quality of life will depend on how we choose to live with, respond to, and manage this inevitable BS of MS.

Let's face it…we've got the perfect built-in excuse to not have any goals, not cross the finish line in achieving a goal, or not even start that race to begin with. We can get stuck and give up, and nobody would fault us for that.   They'd simply say *"Well, you know, she's sick…"* (the *"bless her heart"* is implied) and think nothing of it. But, do we really want to live "less than" because of the BS that comes along with our MS? My guess is that if you've read this far (or even picked up this book at all), then your answer to that, like mine, is NO. (*Brava!*) So, let's talk about how to get moving again when the inevitable BS of MS may overwhelm us and make us feel stuck.

Yes, you are going to get stuck. Even if you've already cultivated a rockstar mindset and have started achieving some "impossible" goals, it's going to happen. And I can assure you that you'll probably get stuck more than once.   But, here's the beautiful thing: You are ALREADY PREPARED for this…What do you do when you get stuck? You (wait for it...) go right to your Must-Have-Rockstar-Toolkit (BAM!)! This is where all of your hard work from Step One comes into play: We created your rockstar toolkit PRECISELY for this situation... precisely so that you don't have to wonder *"What do I do?"* when you feel side-swiped or overwhelmed by the BS of MS and get stuck, and so that you have no need to panic. You now KNOW what to do when you get stuck: You don't panic, and you go right to your rockstar toolkit like a boss knowing that you've got this covered. Then you decide which tools are the best fit for what you need, and you see which ones you can access most easily or quickly in that moment.

Pick and choose your tool(s) by deciding what you think is most applicable or useful to you at the time, given what has caused you to feel overwhelmed or stuck. For example, you may need to reconnect with your vision or reach out to your external support mechanisms. If you need a different or additional tool, you just pick out another one.

There may be times when you feel like you need to do an all-out raid on your toolkit if things feel extreme. If you feel like getting unstuck may require you to use all of the tools in the kit, then use them all if you need them all because that's why they're there. Again, that's the whole purpose of the kit: For you to be prepared, so you're already ready if—No, I should say *when*—this happens to you. And the fact that you've already prepared yourself is pretty rockstar in and of itself, so you should feel really good about that.

The truth is that we all get stuck...even I still occasionally get stuck, but I don't get stuck for as long now. It's how long you remain stuck that makes all the difference. Maybe I'll get stuck for a couple of hours or minutes and then be able to get moving again...so you kind of graduate in your level of "stuck-ness," as crazy as that may sound. It actually makes a huge difference to go from being stuck for days, weeks, or months (Years?) to being stuck for a couple of days, a couple of hours, or just a couple of minutes. And what I want you to do is this: Don't feel defeated or give up if you get stuck…just try to work on getting stuck for shorter periods of time. If you see that there's a stuck mindset that's dragging out, try to tell yourself *"Okay, here's the amount of time I'll allow myself to be stuck"* and pick a time period. Six hours? One hour? Whatever it is, indulge it or wallow in it if you want to, and then move forward when that time period is up.

The problem with getting stuck is that we can't see past it to the other side of it while we're stuck. It's kind of like anything that we have a fear or a phobia about…we stop in that moment when we think the worst is happening or can happen, even if it's just in our mind, and we can't see past it. But, eventually, that moment will be over and you'll be on the other side of it…and you'll start moving again. That's what I want you to think about. Look past this awful-feeling moment to the other side. Remembering that there is that other side is the first step in getting unstuck. And you use the toolkit that you've built to help get you to that other side.

Here's what you do: In order to get to that other side, you must really focus on what you can do to change your state in the moment that you are stuck because your thoughts and feelings in that moment won't allow you to see past being stuck. It's not possible to think your way out of those thoughts and feelings, so you will have to DO something to change your state and act your way out of them. You have items in your toolkit that will help you to do that.

The key is to do something to immediately change the negative focus that your mind has locked onto. One way to bust that mindset immediately is just to start moving physically somehow. That doesn't mean that you have to stand up and walk or do some kind of strenuous exercise because some of us are not able to do that (but, by all means, do that if you can), but it might mean just shifting the position you're sitting in or moving into a different room. If you're slumped over or slouching, sit up straight if you can. And smile, even if you don't feel happy in that moment. Believe it or not, just the act of smiling will change your state. Turn to your simple personal support tools (like listening to some music or some positive audio) to help you change your state while you're deciding which other tools you'll need to pull out of your toolkit. You just need to do something to interrupt the panicked or otherwise negative loop that may be playing in your head.

Even small shifts like the ones above will immediately bust the negative state of mind that you're in and stop that overwhelmed or stuck loop from playing over and over and over again in your head. Your brain cannot maintain focus on that loop and your new activity at the same time, so that's why the first thing that you'll want to do is put your brain to work on something else.

You may also need to revisit the tools that have helped you start creating your rockstar mindset. We've begun taking the first baby step with some of that mindset work earlier in this book. If you're really and truly feeling blocked past what your toolkit can help you with at that moment, then you may be in the throes of a very deeply held limiting belief that really may be hindering your ability to get unstuck. Visit rockstarwomenwithms.com for different resources and community support to help you get unstuck. And of course there are programs and coaching available there that are specifically designed to help you dismantle and defuse some of the very deeply held limiting beliefs that are holding you back not only now, but in general.

VENT ABOUT THE BS OF MS!

JOIN US FOR "BS OF MS RANT" TUESDAYS

Vent and find support

when the BS of MS is

REALLY getting to you

at

www.rockstarwomenwithms.com

A Final Thought

Being up with the bats and computer programmers in the wee hours of the night is good for kicking around deeper thoughts and "even bigger picture" thinking, and I've been doing quite a bit of that lately. I suppose that I truly am on a quest to continually renew and recharge my inspiration in order to keep myself energized and moving forward, and I'd like to help others to do the same. It's so easy to backslide into our old patterns or ways of existing, even when they feel lousy, just because they're familiar (and they're definitely there waiting to welcome us back with open arms). It's especially easy to do that during those times when the BS of MS is feeling like "too much."

I've realized that a goal of being consistent with and staying true to an "even bigger picture" life philosophy helps me to prevent any prolonged backsliding. So, I'd like to end this book with one last piece of advice for you on your journey to live your rockstar life in spite of having MS: In addition to having motivation that's a match

and a vision for how you want your life to look, make sure that you

also have an "even bigger picture" vision to help keep you moving

forward, especially when things get tough and it feels like the BS of

MS is wearing you down.

My "even bigger picture" life philosophy is summed-up in the well-

known Hunter S. Thompson quote:

> "Life should not be a journey to the grave with the intention of
> arriving safely in a pretty and well preserved body, but rather to
> skid in broadside in a cloud of smoke, thoroughly used up,
> totally worn out, and loudly proclaiming "Wow! What a
> Ride!"[10]

That's definitely my style, so my "even bigger picture" goal is to make

sure that my decisions as I move forward will be consistent with a

"Wow!" result when I look backward one day (I think that a "Wow!"

when I'm looking backwards years from now will feel pretty sweet).

One of my best buddies told me that both he and I will be late for our own funerals, and I think I kind of like the idea of that.

I wish you the best in finding an equally awesome "even bigger picture" vision, and much success in overcoming the BS of MS and building your rockstar life!

JOIN US!

CONNECT WITH OUR FREE SUPPORT COMMUNITY

AT ROCKSTAR WOMEN WITH MS

Share your "WOW" goals,

get help with finding your own

bigger picture vision, and find

resources to help you create a life

consistent with that vision!

Get your FREE BACKSTAGE PASS

at

www.rockstarwomenwithms.com

Notes

1. For those who may not be familiar with the term "BS," it is typically used as shorthand for "bullshit," which is a slang term for "nonsense."
2. National Multiple Sclerosis Society.
3. Quality of Life and Its Assessment in Multiple Sclerosis: Integrating Physical and Psychological Components of Wellbeing. Alex J Mitchell, Julián Benito-León, José-Manuel Morales González, Jesús Rivera-Navarro. Lancet Neurol 2005; 4: 556–66.
4. National Multiple Sclerosis Society.
5. Quality of Life and Its Assessment in Multiple Sclerosis: Integrating Physical and Psychological Components of Wellbeing. Alex J Mitchell, Julián Benito-León, José-Manuel Morales González, Jesús Rivera-Navarro. Lancet Neurol 2005; 4: 556–66.
6. "Women with MS sometimes find it too difficult to apply makeup, fix their hair, or shower...this inability to care for one's appearance can affect women more profoundly than men. People judge women's looks more harshly, so women deal with this more than men." Women with MS. Family, Health, and Happiness. Written by Maryann B. Hunsberger, Reviewed by Jack Burks, MD, Edited by Susan Wells Courtney. The Motivator: Fall 08.
7. *How Do You Feel? Self-esteem Predicts Affect, Stress, Social Interaction, and Symptom Severity during Daily Life in Patients with Chronic Illness.* Vanessa Juth, Research Assistant at the Psychology Department at Syracuse University, Joshua M. Smyth, Associate Professor of Psychology at Syracuse University, and Alecia M. Santuzzi Assistant Professor of Psychology at Syracuse University. *J Health Psychol.* 2008 October ; 13(7): 884–894. doi: 10.1177/1359105308095062.
8. Id.
9. Hendricks, Gay. (2009). The Big Leap. New York, NY: HarperCollins.

10. Thompson, Hunter S. (2009). The Gonzo Papers Anthology. New York, NY: Picador USA.

About The Author

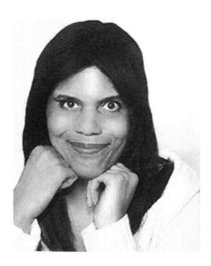

Lisa Cohen is the Founder of Rockstar Women With MS ("RSW"), which is an international community of women living with Multiple Sclerosis who have banded together in mutual support to lead more empowered lives. Having lived with MS herself since 2001, Lisa's vision for RSW is to help women living with MS to live "rockstar" lives, which she defines as living by making active, conscious life decisions rather than auto-pilot decisions by default or resignation simply because of having MS. Rockstar Women With MS advances this vision by providing an active support community and coaching services for women living with MS.

A self-proclaimed "escaped" lawyer, Lisa has more than 20 years of personal experience in life transitions and career change, more than 7 years of experience in supporting others in their dream pursuits, and more than 13 years of experience living with Multiple Sclerosis. Her successful journey to carve out her own rockstar path has led her through the amazing experiences of working in the independent music business, photography/art, and helping to build the nonprofit organization Makeover Your MS. As Managing Director of Makeover

Your MS, Bike MS Champion, and Chapter Ambassador for the National Multiple Sclerosis Society, she is committed to empowering and improving the quality of life of people living with MS. She has a B.A. from Columbia University, a J.D. from Columbia University School of Law, and Certificates in Digital & Graphic Design Production and Digital & Graphic Design from New York University School of Continuing and Professional Studies. She currently resides in New York City.

Connect with Lisa on LinkedIn, on Facebook, or at Rockstar Women With MS.

Made in the USA
Middletown, DE
12 July 2019